A REFERRED PAIN

reflections on family life & cancer

Penny Snow

Patten Press

Newmill, 1997

Published first in 1997 by the Patten Press.
The Old Post Office
Newmill, Penzance, Cornwall TR20 8XN
Tel: 01736 60549
FAX: 01736 330704
e-mail: OldPostOfficeNewmill@compuserve.com

ISBN 1 872229 14 X

Typeset in house at the Patten Press
Printed & bound at The Book Factory, London

Table of Contents

Acknowledgements

With thanks to Doreen Edwards for typing the original manuscript, my husband for his support, our daughter and her friend who played patiently in the garden while I worked, My husband's family and my friends who are such good listeners. Amongst the latter are Sheila and her family, Shirley, Kirsten, Joseph, Annie, Pauline and Terry, my counsellor Sue Brookes, 'James', Thea, John, Pete and Kate. I also thank the writers who have encouraged me, particularly Rosemary and Tina, my friend who made very kind remarks about 'Alice and Katy', the people who cared for my mother, my colleagues at the Family Centre and Melissa Hardie and Ann Dent who had faith in my book.

DEDICATION

For my mother, father, and Susan

FOREWORD

At the age of 21, Penny Snow watched her father wither away -- the victim of cancer of the colon -- unaware that she would go through similar torment fourteen years later as she witnessed the slow painful death of her mother at the mercy of the exact same disease.

A startlingly honest portrayal of deepest emotion, *A Referred Pain* charts Penny's struggle to retain her own identity whilst faced with the financial and emotional responsibilities of caring for a lively toddler on the one hand, and a terminally ill mother on the other. Never far away is her ability to find humour in the darkest of situations, and yet always apparent is the profound effect that the death of a loved one has on the whole family. Confronting the emotions which most people hide deep within their subconscious, this book will be a great help to those who have lived or are living in similar situations, as well as being an enlightening experience for those of us lucky enough not to have been so directly affected by cancer.

Before January 1991, Penny's mother Ann was an apparently healthy woman, well known for her love of life and love of people. I had met her some 15 years before when, after the death of my baby Hannah, she had knocked on my door offering a green plant and as many words of comfort as she could muster. I hardly knew her at that time -- and the fact that she had summoned the courage to face such an unknown situation touched me and our families became close. I often miss the visits she regularly made to our home, which were always accompanied by the words "Hello Sheila, I'm not stopping a minute." and which, much to the good of all of us, usually lasted several hours.

A *Referred Pain* is a fitting title for a book which deals with the anger and hurt experienced by everyone who must come to terms with the loss of such a loving person. It is clear that the physical and emotional pain of cancer is not only felt by the sufferer, but also by those around them -- the loss of what might have been is as strong for the granddaughter as it is for the daughter as it is for the dying mother herself. Penny offers an insight into the frustration, guilt but also the deeper self understanding which is borne of this disease.

I encouraged Penny to write this book because I was acutely aware of what she had to offer other people. Over the months, I saw that as she confronted the emotions she had been previously unable to accept, she gained an inner peace which evades most people all their lives. I hope this book has an equally beneficial effect for all those who read it.

Sheila M. Green

Introduction

Several people encouraged me to write this book and I am very grateful to them because there were many times when I wanted to give up. The emotions writing faced me with were, on occasion, almost unbearable and I became frightened. I was writing about something which had happened in the recent past but reliving the painful memories through writing made me look closely at those years and sharper images began to emerge. I could see more clearly the awful physical deterioration which cancer causes and I realised what a confusing blur everything had been when we were living through it. I also saw that death was an ugly business that went far beyond the physical. A slow death enables those involved to talk through things in a way sudden death doesn't allow but it also puts people under tremendous pressure. What is said or done at any one time may not be pretty. Death isn't always the wonderfully reconciling process often portrayed. Now I am at the other end of writing *A Referred Pain* I feel it has helped me enormously with my grief, anger, sense of loss and my fear of cancer.

This book covers a period of three years, from when my mother was diagnosed as having cancer until her death in

1993. It wasn't the first time I had faced cancer because my father had died with the disease eleven years before. But it was the first time I had been the prime family carer and it was extremely difficult. Unfortunately, as with many carers today, I entered the job having two others already. I worked in a Family Centre and was the mother of a two year old girl. I hope the word 'unfortunately' doesn't sound insensitive. I was lucky to have paid employment which was enjoyable and however arduous the job, I will always feel very privileged to be a mother. What happened to me when becoming the carer of a terminally ill mother, though, was that after some time, I believed I was not doing any of these jobs adequately. Now there seems to be a great pressure on carers, who themselves are trying to support their own families financially and emotionally. In the days of large extended families, some of which were at home the whole or at least part of the time, this was not as much of a problem.

As with being a parent, guilt quite often plagued me in my job of assisting my mother, because my own needs seemed so insignificant compared to hers. Through counselling, I came to understand how suppressing my needs did little, ultimately, to help the person for whom care was required. Time for myself was an essential ingredient if sanity and energy were to be preserved. It was okay to laugh and to have fun during those years. A sense of humour can see us through dreadful things.

Revealing the cracks in my family's life has also been difficult. Admitting that everything is not always 'fine' is obviously not easy and I am especially grateful to my husband for being kind and understanding about what has been written. Like my parents, in a different way, he has shown much courage. Apart from Sheila Green and Sue Brookes, the names of everyone involved have been changed to protect their identities, and I greatly appreciate the support they have given in allowing me to write about them.

Some time has passed since I began to write A Referred Pain. If I were to start now, I think it would be a more detached observation of grief. Time, of course, has allowed me to see certain things differently but I feel that the recording of events at the time they happened or soon afterwards, has its own value.

The appendices are pieces I have written which are directly related to the events in *A Referred Pain*. I have found writing, perhaps, the most helpful therapy. It is not only a release but a way of seeing myself and others more clearly. Sometimes I wrote about things I thought were 'got over'. 'Alice and Katy' is such a piece, written after the birth of a friend's daughter when I realised how little recovered I was emotionally from my own miscarriage. We often grieve over what might have been and imagine what our lives would have been if we had not suffered such a loss. In a similar way, 'When I grow up' considers this. 'Kowloon in the Kitchen' reflects on what life could have been if less time had been spent on matters that, at the time, take on enormous importance but which, when faced with death, are insignificant. 'The Carer' is about feeling helpless and bored, while 'Black Bin Liners' tries to suggest the emptiness of material things when the owner no longer lives.

My hope is that this book helps other people who are facing or who have faced similar situations.

Penny Snow, 1997

It wasn't until I was thirty-six that I realised how profoundly cancer had influenced my life. Most of the time I felt empty rather than bitter, but I often wondered how my life would have unfolded if my father hadn't died during my student days and my mother fourteen years later. This double loss left me with a husband I had married before graduating from University and a five year old daughter devastated by her grandmother's demise.

I had grown up with my parents in an affluent suburb of a busy city. We lived in a detached house like the one drawn by children, the square on top of which sits the triangle, and the long, rectangular chimney perched precariously to one side. During cold, winter evenings or on my Christmas Eve birthday smoke would whirl out of the chimney. There was even the long garden which stretched before the house with a pink blossom tree on the left.

I had enjoyed a close relationship with my parents, but unlike the house, it wasn't idyllic. Sometimes angry and despairing, it was a closeness that shared merriment and warmth and snuggling up in bed when wardrobes resembled monsters.

The realisation of the pivotal place of cancer came to me in my mid-thirties. When my father died I was just twenty-one, in love, and enjoying days where my main responsibility lay in delivering essays on time. The horrors of my father's emaciated figure, his bony nakedness linked to a catheter seemed a long way away once I had returned to my studies and the marital bed. Later, at the age of thirty-six I knew these images had never left me.

* * *

1

My father had been handsome, tall and dark as well. An elegant man who retained a slim figure into middle years, his features suggested Middle Eastern origins. His refined way of dressing heightened an aloofness which belied his humour and sensuality. Quiet and pensive much of the time, he was also something of an entertainer and was often found dancing round our house with my mother, cheekily trying to distract her from her work. This was usually met with weak protestations from his wife, who secretly revelled in the attention and mirth.

Despite the inevitable mundanity of married life, my parents seemed able to hold on to some of the vitality of a new relationship. Frequently they could be found holding hands in public places, giggling about this or that which had amused them hours before.

He was a kind man who listened sympathetically to colleagues, friends and to me, when, in teenage years, I sometimes found him more approachable than my mother (probably because my mother's role as chief disciplinarian had been carefully mapped out for her). He ignored his cancer, the diagnosis of stomach bug believed, and dutifully took Milk of Magnesia, even when the sickness refused to abate and nearly caused injury when driving. By the time he was operated on, the cancer, originally located in his colon, had spread to the liver, leaving little hope of much life. When he finally wanted to know the answer to the terrible question, inescapable for him, of 'How long?' he asked my mother to confront the consultant. When the answer came back, 'a few weeks' he was sitting in our garden, hoping for what he would never achieve, a suntan.

Those few weeks were harrowing as my mother and I, helpless in our exhaustion, watched the slow disintegration of my father. It was if his body had evaporated. His shirt sleeves appeared to have no arms in them, the cuffs fell over his fingertips and the collar could have wrapped itself twice round his neck. There was no bottom to fill his trousers which, when we forgot to pierce a new hole in the belt that pulled them together, dropped to his ankles, cutting short his scuffles round the house. Weary, he stood waiting for them to be pulled up.

2

I had never seen anyone like this, and wondered how much suffering had to be tolerated before certain death came. It seemed wrong that a parent should suffer such indignity in front of his own child, particularly when old age was nowhere near. I felt a deep pain inside watching, and tried to remember him as he was before. It had been said to me that it was worse for those looking on, but one evening, as I saw his body take nearly three quarters of an hour to climb the thirteen stairs to his bedroom, I didn't believe it.

On the last morning of his life, an August Bank Holiday Sunday, we sat quietly in the kitchen, as upstairs in his room the district nurse made sure he was clean and comfortable. Staring into cold cups of tea, we could hardly look up when she told us his death was imminent.

With the help of medication, he had become calmer over the last few days and his weird ramblings had ceased. Now there was a silence broken only by little noises which I couldn't penetrate. Though his body lay peacefully on the plumped up cushions for me to see and feel, he was no longer there for me. I wanted to tell him about the essay I was writing, about who I had seen at the shops yesterday. But there was no point. The only response would have been the stifled rattle in his throat. Soon after, as the warm sunshine of that Bank Holiday came through the window and rested on his clammy hand, my father died.

* * *

My mother wasn't as introspective as my father had been, rather a gregarious woman who attracted many friends. Sometimes outrageous in her behaviour, she would dare to say what others thought and was ahead of her time in much of her thinking. Her own childhood had been constrained by a repressive father and the norms of a peer group who had settled for dutiful sex and a regular perm.

She was often described as 'different' for there was a passion and a wildness in her more suited to the clifftops of some craggy coast than to a neighbourhood coffee club. She was more roundly featured than my father, latterly with grey hair she described as being 'just mousy coloured' before ageing overtook. Her smooth skin resisted wrinkles to the end of her life. Any frustration she felt was shown by angry outbursts, sometimes culminating in the untimely demise of a well loved object lying in her path.

My mother's artistic side remained undeveloped because childhood measles had left her sight impaired. She belonged to an age that contented itself with putting any resources the family had into the education of the son. Perhaps her greatest achievement, though, was her ability to listen to others without judgement or bias. 'You can talk to Ann about anything', it was said.

This listening quality didn't show itself fully to me until my father died, but I knew then that I could discuss almost any subject with her in a way not open to many children. She taught me from an early age that humour was an invaluable survival tool. Our conversations about my traumas often ended with both of us in peels of laughter, cackling until our stomachs ached. She would be a very difficult person and friend to lose.

I think my mother had known for quite a while that something was wrong, but had tried desperately to eradicate such thoughts from her mind. She had the same symptoms as my father, but not wanting to know, she ignored them -- much as he had done. There is a courage in most of us which supports the theory of early diagnosis being the key to a cure. But often this can fail us at 2 o'clock in the morning when, overcome by pain and nausea, the darkness offers little hope. Protective of both my daughter and me, she was also frightened of what her death would mean to us.

When my mother rang to tell me that she had a tumour, I was cutting out an article from a newspaper. In my disbelief I continued to read the clipping while listening to her distant voice. For the first time in my remembrance, Ann became the child again, desperate for some reassurance. I found it difficult to give: the words were said but they lacked conviction. It was hard for either of us to be optimistic with the memory of my father in the back of our minds. Ann's cancer was located in the same area as his had been.

4

The most shocking aspect of this crisis for me was my own complacency. I could see it now, but why, when I had gone through all this before didn't I read the signs? Not only my mother's physical symptoms, some of which she had kept from me, but her undoubted fear had been there for me to see. If only I had shown the courage to question her more. My mother's complaints about a 'poorly tummy' had frequently been related to me when I was nursing my own two year old, so perhaps this had anaesthetised me to the impact, marking it down to a 'bug' not unlike my daughter's. Sometimes she had bemoaned a bad night over the phone minutes before I left the house for work and I dismissed the thoughts, irritated by being delayed for a 9.30 appointment. Of course, I didn't want to believe it because I didn't want my life to change.

The same evening, after her morning phone call, I wrote to her. Even then I continued to write about other things, 'By the way, Clare's enjoying ballet,' I ended. It was January 1991. At this time I had been married for eleven years and had known my husband, Stephen, four years before that. We had studied in the same city, about a hundred miles from both of our separate home towns. By the time our daughter Clare was born, we had been married for several years.

Stephen shared many of my father's attributes, probably the reason why I had been attracted to him. I married him only a few weeks after my father's death. Physically, there were similarities, though Stephen had lighter features. He, too, was quiet and found expressing emotions all but impossible. When these did emerge, they often did so in angry outbursts, discouraging any response. At other times, he showed great understanding and there was a kindness and tolerance towards my own idiosyncrasies. We lived, and still do, in an old terrace house which has plenty of rooms for each family member to express individuality, but only a tiny garden. Space away from each other is more effectively obtained , therefore, in the winter months.

Motherhood had not come easily to me. I was not prepared for the sheer physical exhaustion, and was quickly made aware of how cerebral my previous existence had been. The emotional giving was new to me on the scale required. I had to learn quickly that as a mother I always came second, and that extensive arrangements had to be made if I went out with the baby -- because you had to take practically the whole house with you -- or, if I wanted one of those precious trips out on my own, could her father babysit? If not, who could? This was when a price could not be put on the head of a granny! 'Children rediscover their parents when they have children of their own' a friend had told my mother, and I had to admit this, however grudgingly. In a society which does little to support the struggling young mother, a granny was a valuable commodity.

After Stephen came home from work I told him about Ann's tumour. He was obviously shocked and stood motionless as I circled around him. "It's a tumour, a bloody tumour," I screamed. By now tears flowed down my already flushed cheeks and I glared at him, sure it was his fault. I hurled abuse in his direction, saying anything that came into my head because I felt so much anger. It felt unfair, the sheer injustice of it. He mumbled a few words, reaching towards me but I walked away, too agitated to accept comfort. I paced around because stillness offered no peace. Movement gave me some control, it made me feel I was doing something. It also meant I didn't have to think. I could arrange the airing cupboard, re-arrange it, then re-arrange the re-arrangements. T-shirts on jumpers. Jumpers next to knickers. No! jumpers next to trousers. Trousers next to knickers. Much better. Why didn't I think of that before?

"Why don't you sit down?"

"Because I don't bloody want to."

He offered a cup of tea which I accepted without thanks. It was warm and comforting and it did at least make me sit. He put his hand out, knowing that anything he said would have been wrong. I wouldn't have known what to do, either, if it had been the other way round, but I was still irritated by his presence. So many thoughts were running through my head that he seemed little more than an interference. With a desperation I had not felt in a long time, I

tried to organise my mind, tried to think what the conse-
quences of Ann's illness would be on the three of us. Unlike
the airing cupboard, my mind would not be tidied and
images of my father refused to melt away. I could not
conceive that my mother would finish her life in the same
way. My mother looked so healthy. It was unimaginable.

My father's sallow complexion had at least given us some
warning but the last time I had seen Ann, which was
recently, her eyes had twinkled, her face was pink and
shining. There was no overt indication that anything was
wrong. Cancer had quietly crept up on her.

Stephen found me frustrating because I would not be
helped. Like an animal retiring to a corner to nurse its
illness, I licked my emotional wounds in the privacy of my
bedroom, the door shut firmly behind me. This was met with
anger and resentment, the lines of communication between
us disappearing as the crisis grew. Past hurts were thrown
at one another as the pressure to be strong overburdened
both of us. Stephen and my mother were very fond of one
another and shared similar tastes in music. They sometimes
talked and listened to tapes until late. In her he found a soul
mate and perhaps would find her demise more difficult than
he thought.

In the following few days I went to work, to Clare's
nursery, to the shops but it seemed the certainty of my life
had been snatched from me. Like a deserted raft I drifted,
petrified of the storms to follow for I knew these seas and
dreaded them. We told Clare Granny was poorly -- but not
how ill -- and that I would have to go and see her. It was
the beginning of a time when I would feel my loyalties
divided between my mother and my daughter, and the
wrench would prove terrible.

At the first available opportunity, I drove to see Ann. I
was frightened by the thought of what I might see. It was as
if the diagnosis of cancer might bring an immediate meta-
morphosis, the person no longer the one who had talked a
few days previously. Privately, I still could not absorb what
my mother told me. It defied averages. It was so strange that
the cancer should be in the same place as my father's. I
wanted to rip out the offensive tumour and throw it in the

bin. There seemed a futility about any other action, talking to doctors, operations...the tears blurred the car in front. I slammed on the brakes, vowing never to come in the car again.

Physically, my mother had not changed but her face showed a dreadful fear. Her hands trembled as she gathered mine into them. She was understandably very frightened, and the outward appearances staged for others were now pushed to one side, the lines changed.

I tried to reassure her with remarks such as 'they seem to be acting quickly' and 'things have changed since Dad died' but I was not convinced. She tried to be optimistic, so all I could do was support this attitude. I neither felt qualified nor did I wish to destroy her faith. When I returned home I wrote to her again wishing her luck and sending a picture Clare had drawn at nursery.

Ann's diagnostic examinations prior to the operation were the beginning of indignity for her. She had always been someone who was timid about her body, and therefore, found medical examinations particularly difficult, and would have avoided them at almost any cost. Her operation followed shortly after one such examination which she had found particularly humiliating.

Clare and I stayed with my mother and father-in-law who lived a short distance from the hospital. They provided immediate child-care. The hospital was placed in the centre of the city, difficult to get to and even more difficult to park near. An old hospital that appeared shabbier compared to some, it was one my mother had spoken of often with affection. Finding and reaching it, however, required a level of concentration not readily available to those visiting sick relatives or friends. The first time I went to see her, I nearly did so via the mountains of North Wales, my map reading constantly interrupted by irritable drivers on their way home.

"You could have chosen an easier hospital," I said, exhausted and lounging across my mother's bed, not sure who needed it most. I was convinced I had not been far off spending the night in Wales. We continued to argue, my mother sure of her instructions, but failing to remember that the right turning she had suggested as a short cut was a cul de sac, the getting out of which prolonged my journey by at least an hour. Realising with her usual astuteness that this conversation would lead us down a similar cul de sac, she quickly turned the conversation towards one of the nurses.

"That's Nurse Jones. You'll like her." My mother's eyes lit up. She had the ability to break down many barriers, and that between professional and patient was one. She was forever interested in their lives and spent much time gathering information about her carers so that by the time I became involved, information was usually known regarding the occupation of his or her partner, where they had been on holiday and how many weeks it was before the birth of the next child. "Her boyfriend is a policeman. They are saving for a house." My mother had only been in the bed a matter of hours.

Until her operation, Ann had looked well and continued to live the life of a fit person. When she was wheeled out of the operating theatre, I saw someone I didn't recognise. Completely still, the colour drained from her face, she seemed almost dead. It was the first time in my life that I had seen my mother as ill and as vulnerable as this. It was night-time and the hospital was quiet. It felt as if no-one else was there, only a mother and her daughter. I stared at the corpse-like body in front of me. She was so still.

"Did I look awful?" she quizzed on the following day, simultaneously shocked and pleased that I had been there.

"No," I lied.

"Bet I was a horror," she joked.

"How do you feel?" I asked, scanning all the tubes that appeared from...I wasn't sure where.

"Bloody awful, really," she replied, glad there was someone with whom she could be completely honest. "I'm in a lot of pain."

"Tell them."

"No, I'll be okay. Are you okay? How's Clare?"

"Fine," I said, not wanting to pursue this as talk of anything but the operation seemed irrelevant.

She pointed to a tube which came from underneath the bed and warned me not to trip up over it as this led to her toilet. Such were the conversations between us, a terrible embarassment to someone who had spent most of her life hoping never to admit to being in need of a loo.

"Face it, you're a mess," I teased and smiled, holding her hand. She was in a mess, of course, that I was not sure she would ever get out of. But I also began to realise that the absolute honesty in which I had always believed, was not as easy to put into practice as supposed. I found myself beginning to collude in half truths as she clung desperately to every reassurance. The final acceptance of the truth when it came, was neither from the doctors nor the family, but from Ann herself who understood clearly that she had lost.

When the operation was over, she felt huge relief. She had been terrified not only of the operation but suspicious of anaesthetics. I think, at this point, she believed genuinely that her illness was gone and that she could look forward to many years ahead with her family. She congratulated herself on consulting the doctor as early as she had, remembering my father's delay and at times expressing guilt that she had not encouraged him to seek medical help sooner. Once in the hospital, she felt supported and more able to cope. It was the awful loneliness that accompanied pre-diagnosis fear that had left her floundering.

The hospital visiting that followed was much more tiring that I had assumed it would be. Partly, it was the activity and paraphernalia that went before and after the visits. Bathing and dressing Clare before leaving her with Stephen's mother, the journey to the hospital and the information to be relayed to numerous friends, as to when she would be well enough to see them. When, eventually, other visitors came, they did so in droves, Ann finding herself constantly in the middle of conversations which exhausted her totally.

"I know I am probably being ungrateful, but I told everyone you were coming today and that I would like to see you alone," she finally said one day.

Another equally tiring aspect of hospital visiting, however, were other patients, other noises. No-one wanted to be conspicuous. Whispers, mumbles, half-heard dialogues amused me somewhat but I also reached a point when privacy seemed everything. No matter how considerate people tried to be, I could hardly bear the personal stereos, the portable television, screechy trolleys, pills taken out of bottles, the click/clack of the bed end chart and the seemingly interminable question "Have you opened your bowels today, Mrs. Thomas?"

My mother was probably the worst offender where hospital etiquette was concerned. Very conscious of others, she continually kept the conversation to niceties which, where her illness was concerned, suited her. But when the ward had emptied a little, she changed to a more intimate discussion about my life.

When I rang work to ask for two more days off, they agreed. I felt very lucky with my job. Compared to many women coping with the hazardous cocktail of paid employment, children and sick parents, I was much more supported in my workplace, and I dreaded to think of the pressures that some of my sex struggled under in similar circumstances.

My mother's operation was classified a success, the tumour taken away without affecting any other part of the body. Elated, her sheer joy at having had the fortune of a narrow escape was something to behold. Celebrating her victory, she asked to see Clare who was somewhat bemused by the drips surrounding her Granny.

"They're to help me get better Clare," explained Ann patiently. "This one," she continued pointing to the saline, "feeds me. I am not able to eat like you just now so this is really my fish fingers." Clare stared open mouthed at the drip....the magic of it!

* * *

It was very frightening for Ann to come out of hospital. I sat with her waiting for the taxi and realised how sad and lonely she looked now that she no longer had the surrounds of the hospital bed and staff, the flowers and cards that framed her face for the past two weeks. The idea of her discharge was something she had clung to but like a yearned for holiday, expectation exceeded reality. She had wanted to run from the intrusions of hospital life, but once at home, coping without them seemed to renew her fears. The isolation brought with it a deep sense of how insurmountable the illness was. Sitting alone, there was nothing to distract her from these thoughts.

I thought constantly of cancer too. As life returned to a certain kind of normality, I tried to put it to one side. But it was difficult not to let the thoughts cross my mind several times a day that once more cancer had entered into my family's life. Unaware of it at the time, I was preparing myself for the inevitable conclusion of mother's life. Necessarily this introduced the idea and potential obsession with my own demise.

There was no doubt in my mind that the geographical distance caused me an enormous amount of guilt. It was one of the disadvantages of having left home for another city that when family needed help, considerable arrangements had to be made to be able to offer any. I envied those who could make daily visits for an hour or so. Ann's skills at disguising her situation were very convincing, even though I had become attuned to them over the years. It was virtually impossible for me to know how my mother really was when I could not see her regularly. Fortunately, her doctor was adept at spotting subterfuge in patients after much practice, and could alert me to the fact that she was in more discomfort that she would reveal. The check ups and then the follow ups with the health professionals helped support Ann in a positive way. She gradually began to try to build her social life again, but despite these props, her underlying fears could be detected.

By the summer, it appeared that Ann had achieved a full recovery, the trials of a few months earlier nothing more than a bad dream. She assumed a more confident air, went on holiday and related how she walked barefoot on the beach, the icy waves refreshing her blistering toes. She was thrilled at the expanse and sense of freedom the sea gave her. She believed she had been given a second chance and was not going to waste it walking the perimeter of her house.

Each friend of Ann's I met in those few months after the operation marvelled at her transformation. I became almost tired of hearing how well my mother seemed. Later, when reading back over the diaries for the following twelve months, it was clear that life for us continued much the same as usual.

4 March 1991 -- Ask nursery to take Clare for an extra day next week. (Meeting at work.) Don't forget dentist.

11 March -- Clare - pumps for nursery

14 March -- Drop Clare off 30 min. early (work early) Pumps for nursery. 4pm hair appt.

18 March -- Mother's Day Card! Clare - PUMPS FOR NURSERY!!!

22 April -- Evening - canvas (Local Government Elections)

24 April -- Canvas

2 May -- L.G. Elections - lifts?

7 June -- Weekend - London - Mum & us

14 October -- Discuss Christmas with Stephen

1 November -- Mum's birthday

18 December -- Pantomime

10 January 1992 -- Work-Reviews

15 January -- Clare's B'day party?

8 February -- Clare's B'day

17 March -- Clare's ballet exam

And all this time the cancer in my mother was growing again.

I remembered the visit to London. It had been a hot weekend and I thought if there was meaning to Ann's recovery it was to see her grandaughter's naked bottom bathing in the cool waters of Trafalgar Square. Clare had mischievously sat full clothed in the fountain's pool and then had to remove all she was wearing. So repressed had Ann been all her life about what had been termed 'the nether regions' that she revelled in the delight Clare exhibited with her own body by enjoying the naked freedom and totally disregarding the hundreds who surrounded her.

I noticed when reading the diary that apart from that weekend, no others were marked with extraordinary activity. I recalled vividly the restrictions I had placed on the family over the period of Ann's illness. "What if we go abroad and something happens?" had been my constant refrain. A normality had settled in but only of a kind, and a kind that eventually would confine our movements not just to within the country but within the street. There were hardly any references in the diary to my mother or the numerous visits made to her. It was as if it was so major a part of the year that reminders were rarely necessary, and time spent with her was assumed.

By this time, I had begun to feel that personally I was not succeeding particularly at anything. As the end of my mother's life imperceptibly drew near, I had become confused as to what role I was trying to fulfill. Everyone seemed to be depending on me: my mother for comfort and the continuity of reassurance, my husband for help toward our financial commitments, and my daughter for motherly support during her first year at school. What I yearned for was to depend on another.

* * *

The cruelty of cancer is its recurrence.

I could not erase the memory of my mother's face so overjoyed after the operation. "It's all gone, they've caught it in time. It's gone." She had beamed and I had found myself swept along by her optimism. Now that they had discovered the cancer was there again, I realised how little thought had been given to what it would mean to all of our lives if it did re-occur. We had lived with it, feared it, and subconsciously accepted its inevitability but somehow we had carefully by-passed the practical implications of its return. Like victims of a burglary, we had acknowledged the possibility of such an event, but the video was a loss we were unprepared for.

My mother had suffered pains in her legs for some while, nausea from time to time and an ache in her side. When she

14

could not ignore the discomfort any longer, she cried on the phone to me, frightened that the cancer had come back. Even the slightest cold was met with suspicion and sometimes I lost patience while secretly understanding her apprehension.

After some persuading, Ann had gone to her doctor and been referred to the hospital. "I'm afraid the cancer has recurred," explained the consultant. She was told that the cancer had not been entirely cleared before, and that quick action would be necessary. A course of chemotherapy was offered.

Comparisons with my father were now inevitable and he started to creep into our conversations. What had previously been taboo gradually became the subject of our discussions. It was difficult to avoid "Why us?"

With people generally but with doctors particularly, Ann was deferential. Belonging as she did to a more submissive generation, she wore her 'doctor knows best' badge with pride and duty, being an integral part of her personality, she was never someone who threw medication down the toilet. There were many times when I would have welcomed more information, but Ann's inability to 'worry the doctor' was frustrating and once again, distance proved an obstacle to effective communications on a regular basis.

A course of chemotherapy did seem the only avenue to take but this treatment was like a purgatory where body and soul suffered together. The dictionary definition of purgatory somehow suited my feelings: 'a place where souls of the dead undergo punishment for their sins before being admitted to Heaven.' It did feel as if we were all being punished. My anger was great on behalf of the loss to my daughter whose first years with such an adoring Granny had been so precious. I thought of the times when Clare and Ann would have enjoyed walks together, talks together, gone on holidays together, perhaps until Clare's teenage years. But there I had to stop thinking because the images were unbearable.

* * *

15

In the spring of 1992 when daffodils were appearing in windows and on hillsides, Ann's chemotherapy began. She went to hospital once a fortnight and spent the day there, sometimes the night as well. The therapy was killing not only cancerous cells but healthy ones with them.

As always, Ann found a funny side to her ordeal and unravelled a cheer which I would have found impossible. True to form, she needled nurses for information on the consultant, Dr. Williams, and soon had gathered all the necessary details. One boiling hot afternoon Ann admitted on the telephone to me that she found these visits to the hospital enjoyable. The atmosphere was friendly and her sense of isolation left her. It was being in the company of others in a similar position that Ann found so comforting and reassuring. There were others suffering too, she was not unique.

Ann's side effects were not as severe, compared to my father's whose chemotherapy had left him attached to a vomit bucket what seemed like nearly every waking minute. She did complain of feeling 'knocked about a bit' and the apprehension was terrible. Her fight for life became more exhausting, the confidence which had originally taken her up after her operation was gradually replaced by a timidity. She was fearful of anything which might interfere with the therapy and began to withdraw from people and places. When she did venture out, she was cautious. Often her hands shook and tears were never far away.

Sometimes she tortured herself with questions about what she had or had not done to have brought this situation about. No matter how often she was told otherwise, an element of self-blame was always there. Her life revolved increasingly around the hospital. It gave her life and she was terrified of being too far away from it. She did not show her fear to the doctors on whom she depended so totally, keeping as jovial as possible for them. But she rang me when the side effects were bad. I then rang Dr. Williams who in turn told me to tell Ann to ring up if she was worried. This Ann would do, feeling she had been given permission.

* * *

In June 1992 I was in the early stages of pregnancy. In a way, I felt I was both succumbing to social pressure and an inner guilt about Clare when I became pregnant for a second time. But it was also about something else. There was something life-affirming about the conception. As family members followed one another into cancerous graves, my desire to prove to myself and others that I was capable of being quite literally the bearer of good news was increasingly important. I feared a reputation as the owner of a sad life. Having heard this said of others, I was determined this would not be an appraisal of my own.

Pregnancy, in the present circumstances, would also be a diversion. In my mind, babygrows could replace coffins while tiredness and bouts of sickness offered up as reasons for death-bed absenteeism. For a time it worked. For much of the short duration of the pregnancy, conversations between my mother and I concentrated on the impending decoration of our spare bedroom, successfully putting to one side chemotherapy. It gave Ann something to look forward to, and though Stephen was worried about the financial implications, he was generally pleased as well. Outside of cancer, this had to be the main subject of discussion between us for some time. But Stephen also, long before I did, understood the digressionary meaning of potentially adding to our family.

At the same time, a friend of mine whose daughter was of a similar age to Clare revealed that she, too, was pregnant. We indulged in many and excited phone conversations about our mutual predicaments. For the first time in a long while I felt life for me held more than the care of a dying person, and this filled me with a certain sense of anticipation and pleasure. Partly because of this, when I miscarried shortly thereafter, it felt doubly cruel.

To begin with, there was a teaspoon of blood; I was told this was quite common and that I should just rest for the next day or so. Though physically I could rest, books and

17

videos were readily available, my mind buzzed incessantly. Friends tried to reassure and the word 'miscarriage', like cancer, was carefully avoided. But two days later I finally miscarried. Stephen was a good support, better equipped to cope with physical rather than emotional pain. I clung to his arm tightly as my belly ached and our baby came away from me.

Once I was in the hospital, the radiographer seemed to take a distant and scientific approach in telling me what had happened. "If you look on the screen, you'll see it was two eggs and they're both disintegrating." I was so distraught that I could hardly absorb the fact the the pregnancy had been a twin one. It seemed an insensitive way to describe the demise of two potential lives, but probably this was her own way of coping with the condition facing her on a screen, rather than in the flesh.

As the anaesthetic for a dilation and curretage put me out, I wondered if this was what death was, a sleep you have no control over which carried you off into peaceful oblivion. Later I wondered what had caused the loss of the twins and felt guilty and inquisitive about almost everything I had or had not done for the past few weeks. But to this day I am still not sure if I have grieved properly for these lost children. I think it strange to imagine myself as a mother of three, and have wondered if they would have looked like Clare or had her personality. Nevertheless, having to take things as they came, once the physical pain had gone away, I once again focused on my mother's cancer. New life was not to be. I would have to find another distraction if Ann's continuing predicament was not going to preoccupy my mind completely.

The miscarriage could not have happened at a worse time, coming as it did only a month before Clare started school. As separation piled upon separation, I began to wonder what or who I would have left. I was only too aware of the irony. When Clare had been an infant, school had been the incentive, the light in the tunnel of active nights and interminable days when I felt propped up by the push chair I always seemed to be walking behind. Trundling aimlessly round the local streets I would count the minutes until Stephen arrived home when I might, if lucky, be treated to a conversation.

"When she goes to school I will have an hour to myself," I had always promised myself. And an hour was all I would have liked but somehow it remained elusive. Like the arm I cooked and changed nappies with, Clare was a part of me. I had not realised how attached to this limb I had become. My part-time job had meant that on days when not out at work, I had been with Clare. Now, the six hours in those days without her seemed a long time. Colleagues reassured me.

"You will love it," they stated. "The luxury of a bath during the day" one had suggested, "a good book", said another enviously, but I had remained unconvinced. So dubious was I of its potential that I began to view Clare's first day at school with a dread I had not experienced previously. Her nursery had been such a cosy place. The staff there nurtured her from nappies to numbers, and as I thought of its comfy sofa provided for weary toddlers, I couldn't help thinking of school as an uninviting place. Perhaps it was my own memories of my first day at school. With no experience of child-minders or nursery prior to school, it was the first time I had been separated from my mother. I still remember scrambling over an old wooden desk, screaming for her as she left the classroom. Clare had been looked after by others, had experienced nursery and had an altogether gentler introduction to school life. I soon discovered that most of my fears were unfounded.

School holidays were a new phenomenon to us both. I imagined them filled with slides and roundabouts, films you remembered from twenty years ago, run & re-run, and rainy days when, helpless, you watched the transformation of your house into Teddy Bear's picnic. As it happened, such treats were sparse during Clare's first half term holiday. By the middle of the week, laden with prepared food, and enough pens and paper to supply a class of forty, Clare and I drove up the motorway to visit Ann, who was in hospital having more chemotherapy.

✳✳✳

I had not been with my mother when she was having this therapy before, though she had been going for some months. The pressures of being a working mother were considerable, of course, but I could have had time off. Clare's school did have an After School club which could have been used during the week. But, it was really my inability to accept what was happening to Ann that explained by absence. No euphemistic phrases could disguise the yellowy complexions of those gradually disappearing beneath their bedclothes, their thinning bodies unable to take sips from the water passed to them by relatives powerless to do anything else.

Entering the hospital tentatively, I was trying simultaneously to cope with both my own and Clare's fears. There was a fine balance to be struck between being overly-protective of a five year old and giving information in a way that hindered rather than helped. Ann wanted to avoid most of all the arousing of feelings in Clare that her Granny had just decided to stop playing with her, or did not want to see her any more. The sanitised smell in the hospital hit us as we entered and the hustle and bustle of the ward disallowed any further time for reflection.

Ours was a surprise visit this time, so when Ann's round face beamed at us, and she squealed with delight when she saw Clare, the fears, the smells, the noises fell away. My mother and Clare looked at a drawing Clare had made of Mrs. Evans, her teacher.

Dr. Williams adjusted my mother's box of medications which, like a personal stereo was attached to her with a wire. It held a drug which hopefully was killing some of the cancerous cells. He was a man of infinite kindness and I remembered how he gently untangled Clare's pigtails from Ann's wire when it had somehow wound itself around her.

"We don't want you mixed up in that, do we?" he said rhetorically, stroking the top of Clare's head.

By November of 1992 Clare had settled well into school life, her teacher sensitive to the needs of reception children. One day Clare looked at me earnestly. "Mum, I had to tell Mrs. Evans something today." Cautiously I asked her what it was.

"Yes," she continued, "I was looking at the goldfish bowl and I saw that Sid wasn't swimming around. I said 'Mrs. Evans, I think Sid's poorly.' The whole class stared into the bowl. Then I said, 'Mrs. Evans, I don't think Sid's poorly, I think he's had enough. Really, I think he's decided to die."

My mother was always pleased to hear what Clare was doing at school, but ever the worried mother herself, she spent much time worrying about my increasing commitments. She was of a generation which didn't have to balance family and work quite so finely. I could see why she was concerned because she saw that I could not relax wherever I was. My relationships with those close to me became far more successful over the telephone than they were face to face.

*＊＊

I began slowing down until one day I came to a halt. I lay on the bed, feeling heavy and in pain. I was angry with my body which had become a burden, and the more I believed it had failed me, the more I ached. Every minute of the day I seemed to be obsessed with one discomfort or another, leaving me drained and unable to throw myself into any activity.

I answered such questions as "How are you?" with the obligatory "Fine", knowing that formula questions and answers did suit fine, because I feared any other response. I had to keep going, but also realised something had to done if my mother was to be supported. I was looking after everyone, listening, working, cooking, travelling, nursing.

I continued to lie down. "Sod you," I whispered, half hoping my mother could hear. I was fed up with having to cope with this alone. Suddenly I had a desire to phone a sibling, wherever he or she might be. Was it really true that my mother had been advised not to have any more children after me? I smiled at my self pity for there were many aspects of being an only child that I secretly enjoyed but found difficult to admit. Years of "that must have been lonely; do you miss having brothers and sisters?" I didn't think so, based on the sibling rows I had witnessed. "I expect you were spoilt," instilled in me a feeling that this must be a dreadful predicament because everyone said it was.

Firstly, I had to do something about my leaden body because I slowly rolled off the bed in the firm opinion that the absence of a zimmer frame in the house was, at this moment a significant deprivation. Was this me? I knew I did not want pills, prescribed or otherwise. I could not afford therapy but it was becoming increasingly clear that I needed someone, not something, to get me through the last few months of my mother's life.

I had to look for someone outside the family because Stephen and I were too involved to be helpful to one another, and I was searching for an escape. Home was mundanity itself. It only served as a reminder of the daily traumas.

James was my father, though at the time I did not have the clarity of mind to see this. In the same way as I saw myself as the 'abandoned child' and felt a deep sense of rejection, recovering little since my father's death, I was to become in relation to James 'the rejected friend'. But, his entry into my life at this point was strange yet immensely reassuring.

The child again, I could look to him for a resolution, like I had with my father when I found maternal sympathy wanting. Then I had experienced my father's broadness of mind, an understanding of something less than perfection which I now rediscovered in James. There was the same freedom 'to be as I was' and I sat back and relaxed in his company in a way I had not with anyone for some time. He was my refuge and as with any haven he felt like a safe place where I could slump and let the past week drain away. There were no demands, no bills to pay, no teas to get, no tumours to worry over.

Physically, James resembled my father, so much that once or twice at a distance, I had the painful experience of mistaking him for the man I had lost some thirteen years previously. There was a girlish temptation to jump up and down and wave excitedly at him, the words 'Come and look at what I've just done' almost falling from my lips. Tall and slim, his movements were elegant and quiet. He even

22

dressed like my father, his clothes graceful, autumnal in colour and similarly to my father, he read with the help of circular brown rimmed glasses which matched both his hair and eyes.

One of the first conversations I had with James was about my miscarriage because he was someone I met not long after. The sensitivity he showed towards my situation and level of understanding was quite compelling and, in my experience, unusual in a man. He appreciated my love for the daughter I had and with him, I felt supported as a mother. Sometimes he commented if he had seen me on the street or in a shop with Clare and there was a delight in his voice at seeing mother and child together.

I was ready, despite what was happening with my mother, to feel a woman again, rather than a child. Clare having started school, I was more free physically of her than I had ever been. I began to take a greater pride in my appearance, safe in the knowledge that they wouldn't be covered in baby food by the end of the day. James helped me feel attractive and it was good to feel that again.

Our conversations together reminded me of debates with my father, when long ago my young, untrained mind had challenged the parental view. I had even then been delighted that his interest in my ideas was genuine. Some things obviously had not changed. Despite a certain cynicism, there remained in me a childlike naivety both my father and James enjoyed, an openness they found appealing. Usually I saw him between visits to my mother during the last six months of her life and these meetings made life more tolerable, at times, even light-hearted. They replenished sapped energy, enabling me to deal with the hurdles which followed. Sometimes I wrote to him. When I did I imagined him reading the words and by so doing, found a fluency I had not known for some time. I thought of him as my diary and took great pleasure in the intimacy.

James' mind was sharp, his face searching and although there was a gentleness in his manner, there was also a disquiet I found attractive. Like my father, he was shy of others and wary of his emotions. So there were occasions in my relationship with both of them when it was difficult to

23

feel affirmed. I shared anxieties and uncertainties with James and though my meetings with him were short and the amount of time I saw him altogether was hardly any time at all, I felt a comfort and understanding from a long time ago. Eventually, we took it in turns to reject one another when fear of our own or others' feelings could only be met with escape. This had often been the nature of my parents' relationship as well.

Undoubtedly I was fearful of my own loss of control. Nevertheless, his rejection, when it came and however understandable, was a shock and painful in its absoluteness. By then I had developed a need for him that I had not anticipated. Like my father he was a kind man who wanted to help, but we had turned from one another when frightened. As with my father, much was left unsaid. But James forced me to see how much I had loved my father and how little I had grieved for him.

In December, not long after I first met James, I went for a walk. It was frosty and the moonlight was beautiful. I remember thinking of my mother sitting as she sometimes did, in complete darkness, with only the moon to light her room. She had passed her fascination with the moon on to Clare with whom she used to sit discussing who lived on it. When I got into the city, Christmas lights replaced the moon and I thought of a holiday we had spent in Amsterdam. In the freezing weather, we had watched the trams, narrow boats and tinking cycles over mugs of steaming hot chocolate. We never stopped laughing and I felt so fortunate to have had the opportunity to know Ann as an adult, only wishing I could have had the same chance with my father.

***

From the time that Ann's cancer recurred and chemotherapy was pronounced the only change of survival, Ann and I began to feel that everything we did together we would probably never do again. At first, it was not openly acknowledged. We talked about things we would do when 'this is over'. It reminded me of conversations between my parents when Dad lay dying at home. From his bed, he could see a line of tall, erect poplar trees. Soldier like, they guarded the house against the sun so that beautiful summer evenings were sombre affairs. At times, frustrated by this, he would quietly make plans with my mother, suggesting places they could visit where the sunshine would warm them until dusk, "when I am better". Of course, they both knew he never would be but it got them through the night.

Now, as anniversaries and birthdays were discussed I began to notice a detachment in my mother, a loss of interest. The continuation of life had all but become an irrelevance. By the time Clare's birthday came, an event in other years keenly anticipated by Ann for some time before, Ann sent me some money and expressed only a fraction of normal interest in what was bought with it: a navy blue jumper and a pair of powder blue leggings.

The Christmas just before Ann's death was therefore particularly poignant. Ann had finished a course of chemotherapy a few weeks before and was advised to have a rest from it for a while. Both she and I knew the likelihood of another Christmas together was impossible but neither of us admitted it. The truth was put to one side as presents were exchanged, both 'Merry Christmas' and 'Happy New Year' carefully avoided. I felt a dull ache, a heaviness that could not be erased by gifts, good food or any patter we might hear on the media. We struggled to be joyous for the child in our midst.

We spent that Christmas at our house. I cannot remember why it was organised in this way. But as the days passed I saw that my mother was making her final visit to the home where her only family lived, where she had cooked many meals and dusted as many corners. This was the home she had daubed the walls with posters when I returned from the maternity hospital. 'Welcome Home, Pen & Clare' they had read, with beautiful drawings of children, animals and flowers that she had spent hours completing.

Her ability always to choose an appropriate gift for someone was another of her talents. It was as if she got inside her friends' minds and could see what they would have selected for themselves. I remember one friend saying the quality of your relationship with someone had everything to do with how genuinely pleased you were with the gifts they bought for you. This same person had finally decided to separate from her husband after the third disastrous birthday present from him. If this was the case, Ann had a special gift for understanding and accepting what others wanted. I had never had to wear embarrassing jumpers as a teenager or had to ruffle ghastly dresses to give them a worn appearance.

That Christmas, Ann and Clare giggled together, putting down carrots and water for Rudolph and 'something a bit stronger' for Father Christmas. Whenever Clare was occupaied or Stephen and I were busy, Ann quietly went to her bedroom and as the days passed I saw the effort required to climb the stairs become greater. Ann clutched her side as she slowly clambered up. One evening, when I was in my room reading, she came in to see me but was struggling for breath.

I felt completely helpless. I urged her to see someone.

"I'll be all right," Ann replied, irritated that I had noticed how disabled she was. Her departure from our house after Christmas was her final departure. Tear-stained, she looked hard at it, concentrating on every detail, because she knew now that she would see it only in her mind's eye.

* * *

In January of 1993, Ann saw her doctor who, concerned about her condition, referred her back to the consultant, Dr. Williams. Previously she had never asked me, but this time she wanted me to come with her. On the morning of the appointment I woke up early, lay in the darkness feeling sick, and my stomach was, as Clare once put it, going crazy. I had to get on that train but I was not at all sure how if this queasiness continued. I breathed deeply, remembering similar sensations during early pregnancy, and went to the kitchen for a cream cracker. Nibbling tentatively, my confidence grew a little as my stomach seemed to cope with it.

Preparing Clare for school and myself for the train, we each only just made it. The cracker and water serving as my feast, I still didn't feel well enough to contemplate a cup of tea at the station. I don't know how I survived the burgers, bacon rolls and chips that seemed to pass me incessantly on the train. I felt so ill.

I was to wait for Ann, as arranged, outside the clinic. Arriving first, I looked around for a while and when that became tedious, opened the newspaper for at least the tenth time that morning and pretended to read. Locked as I had become in cancer and child-care, the enormity of world events seemed an irrelevance. That morning I remember my mother appeared in much better condition than I knew I was.

As we waited, we engaged in an absurd conversation about people we knew who had either died or were dying. It seemed compulsive and the more we tried to walk around this conversational maze the more we seemed to end up in the middle with little understanding of how to emerge. Seeing Dr. Williams once more was a great relief as now the responsibility could be shared. Ann's whole body seemed to be shaking and she could hardly undress herself. He pressed her side and wrote on a diagram. She chatted nervously, mainly about Clare and they exchanged comment on living with small children. But Dr. Williams was quiet. There was no difficulty in seeing there were times when he hated his job.

"I am afraid," he said slowly, "it's in the liver again, Ann. The break from chemotherapy has brought it back."

Ann managed to utter a reply of sorts, "not good news, Dr. Williams?" while now visibly shaking and holding my hand so tightly I thought I would faint.

"No, it's not," he said quietly, "but there is another drug that is fairly new. We can try if you want."

Dr. Williams advised her to read the information on the drug concerning the side effects and invited her to see him in a few days time. She was willing to try anything.

"I have had quite a lot of shoulder pain. Is that connected?" she asked.

27

"Yes, it's a referred pain from the liver," he replied. "It's quite common."

We both stood silent as he left the room. I am not sure I fully understood what had been said at that point. But I remember phoning my mother's GP who started talking about such things as an Attendance Allowance to cover my expenses. Slowly I realised that I was going to have to become more involved. I had to accept that my life would have to change. There would have to be After School Club care for Clare...and my mother's demise filled my every thought.

Apart from the unlikely success of a trial drug, the death sentence had finally been passed. The optimism my mother had embraced for the last three years was no longer a realistic option. We returned to her house and I stayed with her as long as I felt able. In the back of my mind was Clare, one hundred miles away, who I had to collect from a friend that evening. I offered to try and change my arrangements but Ann wanted me to go home. What I wanted, I suppose, was a perfect solution and there was no such thing. I knew that professional help was available to her but that felt meagre in comparison to what I felt she deserved. I wanted to give more but with commitments elsewhere, we had to accept a very imperfect situation. That afternoon, I left a woman sitting alone, terrified that she might not be alive the next day. I have never seen such loneliness.

I was grieving for her before my mother died. She was no longer the person she used to be. The spark had gone and fear and weariness came to replace it. I found myself withdrawing when I was away from her. I wanted to be on my own, to sleep on my own, where I could escape into fantasies and shut off the reality that was crowding in on me. I needed solitude, escaping into the world of a book or film enabled me to cope on my own. But I also needed to talk. Three women, Sheila, a family friend, Sue, my counsellor and a friend in Australia with whom I had regular telephone contact, all listened for hours as I expressed so much anger and fear. But for them, I would probably not have managed to survive without becoming very ill.

I had known Sheila since the age of fourteen. We had been neighbours but we had also become good friends, sharing in one another's losses and gains. When looking after my father at home, Sheila who was also a nurse, had proved invaluable. I had often talked with her until night-time was nearly no more. She is warm, honest with a wonderful sense of humour and makes me feel good about myself. There was affinity between us as both of Sheila's parents had died with cancer. I found I confided in her in a way I used to with my mother, who by this time in her illness, I realised could no longer be there for me. Both Sheila and a colleague from work put the idea of counselling into my head. I had shied away from it in the past, fearful of my ability to cope with it and being influenced by what I perceived to be its stigma. Gradually, however, I was realising that I needed someone to whom I could turn in the city where I lived, someone who understood my situation.

I contacted someone with specialist knowledge of cancer, who was able to offer free counselling support. From the moment we spoke on the phone, I knew I would be able to talk with Sue. It was such a relief to know there was someone to whom I could explain everything and who was there when I needed her. We met weekly, usually on Monday, when I could off-load the traumatic events of the weekend many of which were now spent with my mother.

***

"Sometimes I wish she would have a heart attack," I blurted out once to Sue, feeling guilty as soon as I had spoken the words. What an uncaring person she must think I was, but I had by now accepted the inevitable, and almost dreaded the remissions my mother might have; they only served to prolong what already a very laborious process. Why couldn't she just die? It wasn't fair. Sometimes it felt as if she was hanging on deliberately, testing her daughter's level of caring.

That was it! I thought. I was being assessed. 'Commit-ment to dying mother! -- 7 out of 10 -- could do better.' She was trying my patience until it burst. I wanted to shake her and shake her. How much more did she think I could take? 'Care in the bloody community' -- just how could I look after everyone? Why the hell did my mother always ring at 5 o'clock, just when I was cooking Clare's tea?

"No, I can't ring your doctor now. I'm busy and Clare needs her tea. I do care. Of course I care but I'll care in fifteen minutes. He will be there then. I am not being awkward." I slammed down the phone.

This was too much. I had already been through a ghastly day at work and Clare was screaming at me. Ann would probably die now, the phone call on my conscious for the rest of my life. I rang back but it was engaged, possibly taken off the hook. My salvation was not going to come so easily.

It was unlike Ann. She was usually so concerned about Clare's well-being that coming second to her grand-daughter's needs would have been nothing. The new chemotherapy had not gone well, and Ann was feeling lousy. I couldn't remember the name of the chemotherapy medications or most of the tablets or bottles Ann was given by the doctor. They all served as a reminder of what was happening to her and I really didn't want to know.It was not long before mother decided to give up the treatment. She was too unwell and too tired to bother any more.

For me it was becoming almost impossible to care for a five year old daughter in one city and a terminally ill mother in another. There was also my job and my relationship with Stephen. My doctor had suggested that Ann might stay with us but it was difficult to imagine accommodating Clare's and Ann's needs under one roof: the one running around, the other needing peace. Recently, she had even been asking me to come and see her on my own. She said she would love to see Clare but was too tired, and she broke down crying as she said it.

The gradual parting of my mother and Clare was very painful. "I don't want her to see me looking like this," Ann said despairingly, as she became more jaundiced and her jumpers fell to her knees. Ever protective, her heart ached for Clare, but she had also become self-conscious about her appearance. It was often difficult to persuade her that it was

30

important for Clare to continue seeing her as far as was possible.

It was Ann, however, who wanted to stay in her home town, near the friends that she felt close to all her life. She was over-considerate as well about the demands that were being made on me. She did not want to live with us and convinced herself it wouldn't work. She did not want Clare to feel restricted, and preferred to stay with the doctors she already knew. She was beginning to find the stairs at home a serious problem and though she had good neighbours and friends, I realised that this would soon be insufficient.

Though the train journey to Ann's house was a monotonous necessity, it did give me time to prepare myself for what lay ahead, and I was answerable to no one on the journey. On one particular day, there was an irritating delay, heightened by an apologetic announcement and an offer of soft drinks. This foretold a longer wait than forecast, so I rose reluctantly from my seat and made for any telephone that might be available. A call to Ann's doctor was necessary and would relieve my growing annoyance as I had arranged to meet him at my mother's house.

The buffet attendant looked prepared for war. This was not the first time he found himself in such a situation and was well prepared. He knew the rules and was going to keep to them. Undeterred, I began, "I need to ring a doctor," I said, staring at his mobile phone. I explained my situation, continuing to glance at the phone as I did so.

"Sorry, but you can't use that one," he replied, following my eyes. "That is just for the use of employees." The fact that it was an emergency did not seem to have any affect and by the time I had bought a phone card and queued for the public phone, the appointment time with my mother's doctor had long gone. I muttered some words, the least obscene of which was 'outrageous'. I knew that my anger had far more to do with my own anxieties than with instilling any feelings of guilt in the train staff.

The train remained stationary for a long while after I had finally managed to phone. I thought of myself, like the train, in the middle of nowhere. In the middle of nowhere on this train, in the middle of nowhere in my life. Feeling pulled in every direction I had begun to lose sight of the person being torn. To indulge in self pity felt something of a crime but like losing my name when I married, I had lost a sense of who I was. I looked out of the window. The scene had changed, houses rather than sheep filled the frame. The train was at last moving.

I telephoned Ann's doctor when I finally arrived. He expressed his own concerns about whether or not she could continue to live on her own. His judgement was trustworthy because he was aware of the difficulties of our situation. He would not have wanted to engender any feelings of unnecessary guilt, so when he voiced his opinion, I knew things would have to change and soon. Left alone with her at the finish of our conversation, I felt a certain sense of dread. I was beginning to see the disease rather than the person. Whenever I stayed for two or three days I was so frightened she would die overnight. When I took her a drink in the morning I would shout her name and knock at the door several times before entering. Usually I would put on the radio as soon as I got up out of bed, because then there would still be sounds of life, even if it had ceased to exist in her bedroom.

A few days later, when speaking to Ann on the phone, I asked her what she was doing?

"Combing all my hair out," came the reply.

I was silent.

"Well, its dropping out anyway. Might as well help it along," she continued.

From a woman who had been so sensitive about her appearance, and who had consistently subjected me to a hairdresser's post mortem, these were strange words. But now, there was an underlying acceptance about her situation which surprised me.

I put down the phone, thinking of Ann's comb stuffed with grey hair. Her baldness seemed a long way off but each strand was to quickly fall from her head, as if in a hurry to escape from the cancerous body which held it there. Her hair had been straight, and she had successfully resisted both in middle age and later years, the over curly perm, a not inconsiderable achievement for her generation. But her hair was not neat, rather it bent to the will of the elements, expressing a childlike freedom. Its tousled appearance reflected her character and contrasted starkly with the beautifully well-coiffed wig she eventually acquired. When I first saw this wig, I knew my mother hated it because she kept touching it, trying to encourage a more natural look. After a while, when it was obviously becoming too hot to tolerate, she left the room.

"Won't be a minute."

She went to the bedroom but left the door open.

When I passed the opening, I saw the back of a fragile old woman sitting quietly on the edge of the bed, unable to move. The back was the same as ever, slightly bent and unsure of itself but the head was different. Not a hair on it, it hung low, sad, too poorly to hold higher.

I tried to make encouraging noises about the wig, saying how tasteful it was and how like Peggy Ashcroft she looked -- but she was terribly self-conscious about it and spent a long time adjusting it before she would let the doctor or nurses through the door. She only thought about how ridiculous she looked and how horrible she felt, not harbouring rational thoughts such as the fact that they must have seen wigs before. "What did it matter compared with your health?" I asked dismissively, trying to be supportive. But, of course, it mattered a great deal for a woman to think of herself as bald. And it was this indignity which I am sure helped her to decide that perhaps death was a better alternative.

The saying goes, 'If I had a pound for...' and if I had one for every time my mother told her doctor she was fine, only to ring me minutes later to tell me she was not. There were times when I could put up with this and times when I could not. It seemed a waste of everybody's time and highly irritating when it meant that I had to stop whatever I was doing and take an hour on the phone sorting it out. Occasionally I became very angry and we would scream at each other down the phone. She would ask 'What the hell did I know? Had I ever felt so frightened?' I suppose I hadn't.

I felt let down by my mother. I hated her carelessness, her almost deliberate attempts to destroy herself. I could not understand the way she ate the wrong things, mostly for comfort, but I wondered why she didn't find that elsewhere. She seemed to have learned little from my father's death. As I judged her harshly, similarly I succumbed to the same gastronomic temptations, as tears mingled with chocolate gateaux.

***

I t seemed like a hospice might be the only and the best option. Ann could not shop or cook and though neighbours helped, she did not ask for as much help as she should have done. She needed people to nurse her and simply to be with her. My father had been nursed at home. My mother deserved the same but the circumstances were different. My father had Ann to care for him and a daughter at home on her summer vacation. Fourteen years later life had become more complicated.

My counsellor pointed to the physical exhaustion that would result if I lived with my mother for the duration. She said that the hospice staff would take care of all the physical difficulties, leaving time for Ann and I to talk. I understood that quite often, when people look after a dying person at home, there is no opportunity for grief until sometime later, because of tiredness. Nonetheless, I felt inadquate and couldn't erase the feeling. Even though my mother and everyone else involved agreed that it was the most appropriate solution, the 'appropriate solution' seemed callous somehow. I sometimes resented my other, everyday responsibilities. My mother was not going to be alive much longer and she had spent half her life looking after me.

Then I thought about the reality of caring for my father. It had been hard and they had only just about managed it with the help of nurses and Sarah. A lot of weariness came, not from my father and his treatment, but from the endless phone calls and visits. It seemed awful sounding so ungrateful, because it was lovely that people cared so deeply. But sometimes it was surreal as I handed out what seemed the twentieth round of teas one day, and felt I was hosting the longest party I had ever known.

The weirdness was not confined to home. When Ann accepted the idea of a hospice, after her fears of not ever returning home had been allayed, she asked Stephen and I to look around the local one. Altogether it seemed a ludicrous experience. I wanted to say the rooms looked better than in the photographs, but screaming 'For God's sake, my mother's dying; I don't care what the lousy bath is like' would have been more truthful. Naturally he was trying to be as sensitive as he could, and the tour was not his fault. I maintained the appropriate control, but the piece of theatre continued at Ann's house.

"What was it like?" Ann asked nervously.

"Very nice. You will be comfortable there. The food looks good."

"The room's got a..." (Well, it did have a lovely view) but I stopped myself.

"You don't have to share with many others," Stephen reassured her.

I think she understood that a hospice was the best alternative but I was never entirely sure what she felt about not being looked after at home. Both Stephen and I wished that Ann had been at home for us to look after, but we needed the money from my employment. There will probably always be some lingering doubts about whether or not we could have done more.

The hundred mile rail journey to the hospice occasionally gave me the false impression that it would take me somewhere pleasurable. There was a lack of excitement being closeted with the car radio, which came from the train journey and sharing the travel with others. It reminded me of times, now passed, when I visited a friend in London and could enjoy several days of teas, meals and chatter, interrupted only by a play or a concert. This was only three or four years ago, but those days belonged to another age. When I put away my book and prepared for the inevitable battle between my bags and the sliding exit door, I thought of that friend, now living in Australia. Then as the train jolted to a stop, I remembered that this day ahead had little to do with pleasure.

There was something very powerful about the doors of the hospice because they took me from a world I knew to one that was alien. The sunshine and fresh air I left outside were replaced by a smell and an atmosphere like no other I knew. I could easily have walked through the doors with my eyes closed and known where I was. The kindness and warmth shown to my mother and I were things neither would every forget. The staff took the physical work from me and allowed me to talk whenever I needed, but when my feet passed through the doors I did not feel I belonged. I was sure my mother felt it too because there were times when I looked into Ann's eyes and saw the strangeness reflected there.

It was more restful to be in a hospice than in a hospital, smaller wards and soft lights encouraged a homelier feel. Like me, mother appreciated the absence of everyday worries living at home had not allowed her to forget. In some ways she seemed better than she had for some time. Being in the company of others, always important to Ann, meant that she chatted often with them and the nurses. She began to believe she might return home. In the hospice we could talk in a way we hadn't managed to when she was at home, due to the concerns about her ability to cope. We talked about my father and I cried on several occasions when she told me how proud he had been of me and how much he loved me.

The whole family could also visit. Clare pulled her drawing books out of the Disney backpack she lugged in from the car and chucked them onto the cream coloured bedspread.

"Gran, can I have a drink?" she said in a loud voice. It did not matter that her grandmother was in a hospice; it was still her Gran and she wanted a drink.

Ann, ever concerned about Clare's welfare, began to think of ways they could find one when the little cafe, usually open for visitors, was closed.

"It's okay, I'll go to the shops," Stephen offered.

On his return, Clare tucked in, glad of the packet of crisps though she would have preferred cheese & onion.

"You are going to die aren't you, Gran?" Clare didn't look up, her crimson HB pencil busily colouring in Minnie Mouse's dress. There was a second of silence before Ann's laughter covered her embarrassment and shock at this openness. She ruffled the top of Clare's head whose face was still intent on her drawing.

"Well yes. I am," she said.

An hour later as Clare and I put the finishing touches to Bugs Bunny's ears, Ann offered fruit and biscuits to Sarah and her husband who had joined us meanwhile. We laughed about things that had happened since we had known one another. I remember thinking how strange everyone's hilarity seemed at an inappropriate time.

"How long do you think I have?" my mother asked, laid on the sofa, propped up by numerous cushions. She was quite sallow now. She raised her hand limply, asking for it to be taken. I held it and tried to answer as honestly as I was able.

"I don't know," I said quietly. "I think you will decide." But she had fallen asleep. Coming out of the hospice had been an achievement for my mother. She had regained some strength and a willingness to fight for more life had returned. She became wary of catching colds or the flu. I thought it was something sadly ludicrous to ask people who might have something wrong with them, not to visit. But I respected her wishes and kept away when I could hardly see due to conjunctivitis. After a couple of weeks though, my mother's strength drained away. Her body was thin and tired. A flicker of humour remained and we joked about her asking me to make sure to put on her knickers if she died without them. I replied that I didn't feel very confident about putting a pair of Marks and Spencers best on a corpse, and posed the question, "Do you think you or the doctor will care?" I knew it was a dying wish but asked if she could think of another one.

* * *

After Clare's ballet class, leotard, tights and dainty shoes were thrown into the back of the car. We piled in, ready for the journey to my mother's house. For me it was crucial that Clare's life should remain as normal as possible with as few disruptions to her routine. I blamed myself when Clare had to make sacrifices because of Ann's illness and was often troubled by constantly juggling Clare's and my own timetables.

When we arrived, we entered the house using our own set of keys. There was no smell of food. It wasn't that I expected it but it was yet another grim reminder of the grave reality we faced: the mother, the nurturer, the provider of nutritious goodness had vanished into a past that could never return. Bubbling, simmering vegetables and stews were nowhere to be found. I heard Ann's voice.

"Is that you?", my mother walked unsteadily, but the hug she gave Clare was as firm as ever. "Alright?", she squeezed my hands. There were tears in her eyes. That familiar look of 'What a mess' written across her face with its plastic, cancerous appearance. She made an enormous effort to smile, "Okay, Stephen?" She shuffled with Clare to the kitchen, came back and pressed a Ten pound note into my hand. She asked us to go and get ourselves something to eat as she couldn't cope with the smell of cooking. We gave the money back, telling her not to be silly and went out to eat. Later, we all went out because she felt like some air. As we walked slowly round a local park, I was acutely aware of people's avoidance of us, and the look of discomfort on people's faces when they saw my mother.

Ann was a restless spirit, a person who found the four walls claustrophobic, one who would constantly find things to do outside the home and have friends to see. The immobility of this long illness was all the more unbearable for her to cope with and for me to watch. I felt that we had crossed a boundary that day by encouraging someone to walk out in the open who was in such a late stage of terminal illness.

We sat down on a park bench while Stephen and Clare went for a walk.

"I forgot to take my anti-nausea tablets," she said as she began to heave into an inadequate piece of crumpled up tissue. (She was always in possession of such tissue to be produced in moments of crisis, always reassuring the receiver that 'it's clean' despite a well worn appearance.) I hated this. I couldn't cope with vomiting though equally I felt terrible for thinking of myself in this minor crisis. I ran towards Stephen who was playing ball with Clare by the pond. He was good with illness and had always sat calmly with Clare and the obligatory sick bucket when she had a 'bug'.

"What's the matter?" Clare looked frightened.

"It's okay. It's Granny. She's not well."

I took Clare to a bookshop near the park while Stephen helped Ann . We bought a book which Clare wanted and could later read to my mother as they cuddled up on the sofa.

Some days later, Ann's next door neighbour tried to reach her on the phone. Then she heard a thud. Fortunately she had a key to the house, and when she opened the door she found Ann lying on the floor, laughing. She asked another neighbour to help pick Ann up, a man about my age, who duly lifted her thin body from the floor. Whether or not it was the drugs, everyone generally considered that she could no longer live alone.

By the spring of 1993, I knew my mother's life would not last much longer. The unfairness of it all still weighed heavily. One of the strongest hurts remained that she and Clare would not have each other when they were both much older, Ann mediating between teenage daughter and mother in those difficult years. I recall taking days to choose a Mother's Day card that year. From Impressionist paintings to photographs, blues and purples to orange and yellows, none of the flowery images felt good enough. There were still things that I wanted to talk to her about if she had lived longer because there was still so much I felt angry about: the lack of confidence which she had passed successfully on to me, her difficulties with relationships. But, this was not the time. There is, of course, a good chance if she had lived to one hundred and three, they would still have been left

unsaid, because the time is never right for certain conversations. Nonetheless, on that last card, I thanked her as
well as I was able, for all her support over the years.   She
replied, telling me of her 'gloriously happy memories' and
how she enjoyed the laughs but also how we had managed
to get through the downs as well. How being a mother and
grandmother had been the most important things in her life.

* * *

When Ann went into the hospice, I no longer wanted
to stay in her house, for I doubted she would ever return.
By this time I was spending days away from my own home.
A neighbour, Alison, a woman about my age with two small
children, offered to let me stay with her when I came for a
visit. A warm , lively person who seemed to tolerate a never
ending stream of visitors, she plied me with food and supported me throughout. Despite the difficult circumstances,
I almost enjoyed the times I spent there. I could not help
but feel that there was something odd about living through
a crisis, awful though it may be, which was almost exciting.
Like snow cancelling school, cancer had allowed me to stray
from the tedium of everyday life. But eventually it developed its own tedium and as time went on I began to feel
differently.

It was the double life, the waking up in different beds in
different parts of the country, the constant change from the
role of wife and mother to that of daughter, the guilt
attached to too much time off work, the cancer 'improving'
and 'worsening', the never knowing where you should be
when and seldom being satisfied with the place you ended
up, that finally defeated me. All of these and the exhaustion.

I wanted to go home. I missed Clare, her voice as she
chattered about school. After four days I felt I had been
away long enough, but the hospice doctor thought that
Ann's condition was deteriorating and urged me to stay.
Distressed and confused, I went to see one of the GPs in my

mother's home surgery. I felt I needed to be pointed in a single direction. I did not really know where I should be.

Dr. Howard was an unexpected gift. As with any such present, it was the surprise which was as uplifting as the gift itself. Unexpected, because there was an honesty in this doctor about her own feelings for Ann which surprised me. She asked if my husband was looking aftr Clare. When she knew he was, she urged me to stay a little longer, pointing out that I had the rest of my life with Clare. Then tears rolled, first slowly, then uncontrollably down her cheeks. "I like your mother so much," she managed to say with some difficulty. "I'm new here. She has made me feel so welcome, taken such an interest, even though she must feel so unwell. I always look forward to seeing her." We held each other's hands. I stayed another day, but my urge to go home was so overwhelming that I left when my mother's condition had, once again, 'improved' a little.

I was back at work when a phone call came through from the hospice. "Is that you, Pen?" my mother asked. She sounded distressed.

"Yes" I replied quietly, not knowing what to expect and not really wanting to hear. I was cross because cancer invaded my life every single day. I put my head in my hand, exasperated and tired.

She said she would like to see me as she was convinced the hospice staff were trying to get her into a home and they wanted her money. I felt like crying but my surroundings stopped me at first, then they didn't. Unable to focus properly as my eyes filled up, I sensed my colleagues were no longer talking to each other. It was as if permission for tears had been granted, so they fell. When my nose ran, tissue was provided.

"I can't talk, Pen. They're listening," she continued. "Are you there, Pen?"

"Yes. Who is with you? Let me talk to someone."

The hospice doctor spoke with me, hoping that I could see him as they felt they needed to do a brain scan. The cancer may have spread there. I told him I would up up the following day.

41

My mother was twitching when I arrived. The anxiety I had heard over the phone the day before was now there for me to see. She was muttering to herself, continuing without a pause when she saw me. Perhaps she had been talking to me for hours. "Don't let anyone upset you," she said, patting my hand as she always had done when reassurance was needed. She started to cry. Unable to hold back my tears, I did the same.

"You just need some love," Ann sounded agitated. It was as if she was trying to work out who would replace her for her daughter, something that had been on my mind almost constantly in the first two years of Clare's life, becoming a terrible hypochondriac in the process. I held her hand. I knew I could no longer talk to her as I had done in the past. It wasn't long before she fell asleep.

The doctor explained to me that they were not sure if the deterioration was physical, and therefore wanted to do a brain scan. He said Ann had become very agitated, it could be a number of things, but they needed to eliminate the possibility of the cancer having spread to her brain. In fact, the cancer had not spread in this way, though the combination of her illness and the medication were causing her to become very confused. I couldn't communicate with her well.

When talk to other people was needed, I went to Sarah who lived only a few miles from the hospice. Alternatively I off-loaded onto one of the nurses with whom I had a rapport and who nurtured me as much as she did my mother. I was touched by the way she sometimes phoned me at home to make sure I had arrived safely, especially if she knew I had just been through a distressing visit with Ann. I asked the nurse if Dr. Williams could visit but didn't expect that he would. My mother had thought him God and being an incurable romantic, it seemed appropriate that she should end her life with a visit from a tall, handsome man.

To my surprise, he visited her one Saturday morning when Ann was lucid. Apparently, they talked for some while. I did not see this but imagined her absolute delight at his arrival. Her prince had come and she was now ready to die.

There were rooms in the hospice where tears could flow freely, but on the wards only the most courageous showed their despair. Like the supermarket, no-one wanted to be there but while they were, observed the social niceties. Unable to talk to their relatives who were too ill to hear or understand what had happened when the plumber came yesterday, carers often found themselves confiding in one another. This was sometimes comforting.

When conversation was too difficult, I attempted to sit on the chair next to Ann's bed with my book or a newspaper but was too restless to take in most of what I read. Then I would pace around the hospice, up and down, up and around. There was something nomadic about these wanderings. I had lost my base, my anchor in life was about to die and peace had left me.

Bored with reading about the forthcoming Summer Fayre in aid of the hospice on the notice board, I went back into the ward and checked to see if my mother's glass needed more liquid. As the juice trickled into the glass, I read a card from someone Ann knew. Covered with beautiful flowers in a soft pink hue it read 'Get Well Soon'.

* * *

One Monday I went to the hospice, intending to stay with Ann for the day, perhaps then overnight with Sarah. I expected my mother to be lying motionless as she had on recent visits, leaving me free to read a book, content in the knowledge that at least I was there, a hand to hold. But this time it was different and I was shocked by what I saw.

My bald, frail mother sat alone talking as if she had an audience. Fleetingly, I thought this meant an improvement. Even at this stage, I occasionally believed in the possibility of it. But, as I drew closer the monologue droned on incoherently and the people about whom she was speaking were people I think I was sure she had never met. Horrifying. Perhaps the worst part was that this jibberish was not constant, lapses into normal speech were interspersed.

"Hello, Pen, you look lovely," and for a moment everything was fine again. The well-remembered scenario of tired and hungry daughter arriving on her doorstep, being greeted by a remark indicating acceptance, played again. But this was a scene, not for a weekend, or a day, only for a few seconds before the incomprehensible chat began again.

She let out an eerie giggle. Who was this person sitting next to me?

"John, we had some laughs didn't we?" Who the hell was John?

The giggle became a sneer. She glared at me.

"Oh, it's you," she snarled. I looked behind myself but there was no-one there. Was this anger directed at me?

"I don't know why you had to do that. He was very upset. Have you flown in this morning?" Ann turned her head and talked to the air.

"My daughter lives in Germany."

Who was this person? Upset who? What had I done? I felt my head spinning. I knew I was sitting by the right bed even though recognition of my mother was becoming increasingly more difficult. But now there were two people: the one whose body I could see, and the one who talked. I tried to dismiss it the thoughts. It was the drugs not my mother, but such a drift left me with the same doubts that fill people who have just witnessed an alcoholic rage. Is this what the person really thinks but sobriety prevents honesty?

It was a beautiful day with sunshine and a light breeze. Ann decided to go into the garden to sit next to red and yellow flowers. I remember wearing white trousers, a grey t-shirt and a floppy beige sun hat that day. It was the last time my mother commented on my appearance so it was an outfit I remembered well and never wore again. Ann should have been a fashion designer because she had a good eye and real flair. But the confidence and opportunities had not been there. In my mind I was beginning to talk of her in the past tense.

I sat on the ground next to her wheelchair and looked up at the woman I loved. Ann was still talking and laughing. Even to attempt to join in felt bizarre. Her bald head was set against the sunlight. It was a head I had come to admire for instead of giving an appearance of decay and pity, it represented dignity and courage. I made appropriate noises where necessary whilst remembering other days when we had sat in other gardens, talking endlessly about family, friends, politics. I yearned for a conversation. The madness terrified me.

Ann complained of the cold and I wheeled her indoors, glad of the opportunity to break this up. I made some excuse to get out of the ward and went to cry in a quiet room. The woman I was visiting was no longer the mother I recognised. My instinct was to get as far away as possible from the one I had left. I longed for my home, my daughter's arms and a conversation I could understand. I had only been there an hour but I left and returned home.

The taxi driver spent most of the drive to the station chatting about the virtues of Classic FM. The music, a piece of Mozart, was loud and beautiful but I wanted to shut it off, put my hands to my ears so that I wouldn't be able to conjure up memories of happier times when music excited an already joyous heart. I couldn't get out of the taxi fast enough, hated the small talk and the bustle, the crisp packets, announcements and personal stereos on the train. I hated Stephen when I got home because he had never seen either of his parents as I had seen my mother that day. I loathed the stupid saleswoman on the other end of the phone who presumed to interrupt my grief by trying to sell me double glazing.

"Do you realise I could be waiting for a phone call from the hospice where my mother is dying!" I screamed down the phone.

My only sanity was Clare. I put her to bed and read her a story, a tale about a furry bear. I loved the way her golden hair lay dishevelled on the pillow. I stroked it and snuggled up amongst the teddies while she told me all about school. I could smell the fragrance of her shampoo, so that tonight I imagined she lay in an apple orchard.

45

"Stroke my back, Mum," she said sleepily.

As Clare's breathing deepened, I wondered what world she would enter tonight.

* * *

It was a Saturday afternoon, hot and sticky and we were in the hospice. Ann slept much of the time now, only opening her eyes occasionally and seeming very weary when she bothered. With the little strength she had left she often shook off the sheet, it was so hot. A fan gently whirred on the table near her bed, causing her nightdress to move ever so slightly. Like many nightdresses, it frequently found itself round Ann's stomach. I pulled the sheet up slowly so as not to disturb her. But this aggravated Ann and she pushed it down again.

It was Wimbledon tennis time, and I sat with Stephen in the TV room...watching for a while. Click, click, click, click. The comical turning of the spectators' heads as they followed the ball, able to rest only after the declaration of a point. Click, click, click, click. Would she die this weekend or wouldn't she? Please someone, put her out of her misery. Put us all out of this. Anything but this. Click, click, click, click. I looked at the television and at the spectators enjoying their sport. Even after all this time, I was still surprised at how horrifying the continuation of everyday life was to me and how wary that life was about death.

The day after that, I went with Sheila's husband to visit my mother again. As we walked in, she was being lifted onto a commode. It took two nurses to lift her frail, thin body onto it. "Alright Ann. It's okay, we've got you." they reassured her, while she muttered incoherently. She looked like a tiny old man and I just wanted to take her away somewhere, anywhere, just wrap her up and hug her and tell her everything would be okay now. An inner voice screamed, "I love you."

They lifted her back to the bed. Her lips seemed so dry and she called out to me for a drink. She loved the blackcurrant drink Sarah and Philip brought her, and took a few

46

sips. Her relief was enormous. She looked at me. "Hello Pen." Then she turned her head. "Oh, hello Peter." There was almost a joy there. They were the last words she spoke.

We sat around at home like soldiers waiting for battle. The tension and the restlessness were hardly bearable. We had lived with this pressure for over two years, our emotions stretching elastically, but now so taut they were more than ready to snap. I knew that there would be a call from the hospice that day.

It was a warm but dull Sunday afternoon. The lull in human activity only heightened our nervousness. Clare sat with me on the floor and drew a picture of a house where the garden was lined with yellow and blue flowers. The phone went and startled me so much that my apple juice spilled over my floral skirt.

"I think you had better come up," said a familiar voice down the phone. "She's a little clammy."

I hardly spoke a word in the car. I knew this was it. Something I had wanted to happen but didn't want to happen. By night-time I would be an orphan. I felt already so lonely.

It was a shock when we arrived to find another nurse expressing surprise at our arrival. "Yes, she did go a bit clammy but she's a bit better now."

I could hardly believe what I was hearing. We sat by the bedside for quite a while. Clare, who had not seen her for some time, was horrified at her Granny's appearance. She ran screaming out of the ward, to be calmed by a nurse. They sat quietly in the TV room playing 'houses' together.

Eventually, we went to Ann's house where we decided to stay overnight. We heard nothing from the hospice all night and by the morning couldn't decide whether or not to go back home. Clare was complaining that she was missing school and Stephen was nervous about missing work. The hospice said her condition was stable.

We went to see Sheila and Peter. They both thought we should go just once again to the hospice. When we arrived, we were told she had deteriorated. Her tiny head sunk deep into the pillows, her witch-like yellow face whose mouth was wide open and whose eyes were closed. I held her hand.

It's coldness made me feel my mother was slipping from me...this was the hand of another world, not the one whose warmness always had clasped mine. "Come on, old thing, don't get yourself so upset," she often said. I wanted to hear that again. I wanted to cut off that hand with its gold wedding ring and keep it. Even in its decaying state I could look at it and remember the comfort it had given me. I could hardly look.

"Don't go! Don't leave me here!" I wanted to shout. I kept turning away, I couldn't watch this. Stephen asked a nurse to check her pulse because he could not feel it.

The nurse stood opposite them. "I'm sorry, Penny, she has died," she said quietly.

As Clare's first year at school ended, so did Ann's life. My husband sat with my mother for some time after, holding her hand, while I went to see Clare and to comfort her. Perhaps he was thinking of a special tune, perhaps jazz, which they both enjoyed. Perhaps he was recalling their long discussions late into the evenings... I sat on the wall in the garden and looked up at the sky. It was warm and a soft breeze brushed against my face. All I could hear were children's voices a little way off. I sat quietly and thought of my mother.

Seeing her in a coffin had been the most shocking moment of my life. The awful finality of it. I had not seen my father in one. I had loved him so much but I could not remember whether or not I ever told him in those last few months. I had written to my friend, James, telling him of my mother's death and he had replied how sorry he was, and what a good support I had been to her.

Stephen, Clare and I carried on 'the same', but it wasn't easy. She had been such an integral part of our lives. Clare missed her; it was dreadful sometimes to watch her face when friends rushed to see their Grannies. Stephen missed her, but he wouldn't talk about it. Instead, he became angry like he had done hours after the funeral when he screamed at me in the car over a spilt drink. And there were no crumpled up tissues to mop it up. I despised him then and screamed back at him.

***

The children's voices came nearer. Where were the parents who had held me tightly and snuggled up in that warm bed?

Tired, I looked at the grass below the wall and reached out for my father's arms. I wanted him to lift me down.

Appendices

Alice and Katy

Alice and Katy sat upright on a red plaid blanket, their soft bald heads bent in concentration. Alice liked the furry thing, for whatever it was, it had a nice smile and big blue eyes that stared at her in a crazy sort of way and made her giggle. Katy preferred piling up the hard things, until they got so high they tumbled down and she had to start again. She liked their bright colours but she didn't know why they all had strange patterns on them. Her Mummy sometimes pointed to these patterns, then looked at her and made loud, curious noises. She thought she was supposed to join in, but for the life of her, she couldn't. Well, not quite the same as Mummy. Alice and Katy's eyes stared in wonder at everything they saw around them and they kicked their fat little legs in sheer delight. They enjoyed this part of the day. They didn't have to do a lot. They were placed in comfy chairs next to one another and a strap which made a clicking noise kept them there until they were lifted out again. Mummy held the chair at the top and for a while she completely disappeared out of sight but they could still hear her talking to them. They saw lots of legs and the odd furry thing, looking a bit like Alice's toy, sniffed their legs and if it was cheeky, licked Alice's bare toes making her giggle once more.

Alice and Katy liked to be fed. They loved the warm, delicious mushy stuff that was gently poured into their mouths and especially loved it on their cheeks. Katy liked it on her hands and when their big sister sat next to her, she reached out and made pretty shapes with it on her t-shirt. It seemed to upset her sister who wailed at their Mummy and Katy didn't see her then for some time after. She was only playing.

Alice and Katy loved their sister, even though she got cross with them. She held them, one at a time, stroked their heads and looked at their Mummy to make sure she was holding them all right. Yes, she was, they felt safe in her arms, as safe and warm as when they'd sucked their Mummy's nipples and drank the milk from her breasts.

Alice and Katy died three years ago when they were fourteen weeks old but that was twenty-two weeks before they were born.

When I Grow Up

When I grow up I want to:
-sit with you
-watch you grow old
-listen to you moan about the government
and exchange ideas for a better way
-rest in your arms when the baby's kept me
awake all night or when I've rowed with Stephen
-borrow some money from you
-see you throw your grandchild into the sky
and laugh with her
-give her to you in the school holidays!
-go to restaurants with you
-go to the theatre with you
-go for a walk with you

When I grow up I want you to:
-watch me as a woman, not a child
-watch me with my children
-see me achieve
-listen to me moan about the life I've chosen
-give me advice
-be there when no-one else is

Now I am grown up, I sometimes wish I could be with you.

Kowloon in the Kitchen

When I'm better we'll get away from here. We'll take the car into the countryside, drive to the top of a hill and where there's an opening, we'll stop and admire the view. We'll drink tea from the flask and I'll tell you about the biscuits I put in the cubby hole earlier. And together, we'll just be quiet.

Or maybe I'll take you to places I never did. Never did as there was the future to think about, the bills to pay and of course, there were the children. So our timidity kept the Himalayas in the living room and Kowloon in the kitchen. I didn't even take you to New York, where my carefree spirit had wandered before I met you. I'll stop worrying about all those silly things that don't really matter any more. I'll buy boxes, put them in and label each box, my job, your job, our house, your car, our insurance, my obsessive desire to please. Then I'll tie a silk ribbon around every one and put them where they can't be found. All those things we argued about. The times we rowed and didn't listen. And then we'll disagree about what's truly important because I will love you in a way I never did. And I will love myself.

The Carer

The carer sat reading her book and sighed heavily. She sighed again, leaned back in her chair and let the book fall into her lap. Her eyes gazed upwards at an old, grey cobweb. It flickered slightly. She stretched her legs out in front of her and the shiny paperback slid off her, onto a carpet discoloured a little by numerous spilt drinks. She could hear the breathing from the bed. It was all she'd heard for a while.

The carer looked at her watch. She wasn't sure why. She wasn't going anywhere. She got up and, in a state of mind which settled uneasily between boredom and nervousness, fiddled with the objects on the dressing table. Nothing was new. One or two of them had been there since she was a child. She picked one up. A delicate vase, meant only for a single flower. She turned it in her hand until she could see the triangular shape at the bottom, carefully glued into its original shape. She had dropped it long ago, when everything to her had been a playball. As if to remind her of her previous misdoings, it now fell from her grasp and a muffled thud followed but it failed to disturb the figure in the bed.

The carer stood at the window and gazed onto a world which couldn't see her for the net which came between them. It was oblivious of her anyway. A car parked. A woman got out from the passenger seat and three shopping bags came quickly after. She thanked an unseen driver and proceeded to cart her heavy load to a front door. Three schoolgirls exchanged gossip, chocolate and homework while a man and a woman waved acknowledgment.

The carer walked away and began to make yet another cup of tea. She was tired and hoped the caffeine would help. She grimaced. Its warmth was comforting but its taste peculiar. She wanted it to keep her from falling asleep. Sleep was all she wanted these days.

The carer loathed the quiet. She didn't even want to be here but the funny thing was, that when she wasn't here, it was all she wanted. She wished she could hear voices other than her own. For a while, she turned on the radio and was partially comforted by Mrs. Smith of Stockport asking the panel if her hyacinth bulbs should be placed in strong sunlight. When she turned it off, the carer found the silence even more so. She sighed again and walked towards the bedroom door. Cautiously, she opened it and looked round to see the figure still sleeping.

The phone rang and woke the carer. She ran to get it, fearful its rings would also wake the sleeping figure. It was her daughter, who rang to say goodnight. She sounded so far away. Everyone sounded far away. She put the phone down and the silence resumed.

The carer paced aimlessly round the house, a house that, before long, would no more open its doors to her. A house that would soon hear another story.

Black Bin Liners

Black Bin Liners
That fill your house
Filled with your things
From long ago

Black Bin Liners
That tell of times
When together, we strode along
The coastal path,
That funny hat
Those awful wellies

Black Bin Liners
That clatter with the cutlery
Upon which stews were served
That clank with framed photos
Slightly out of place
Revealing others underneath

Black Bin Liners
Soft and squidgy with piles of jumpers and scarves
Worn on trains, in theatres
And every school concert
I put them to my nose
And can still smell you

Black Bin Liners
That carry your candles,
Ornaments, books
And pictures painted by friends

Black Bin Liners
That tell of your life
But how can I recapture
Your warmth and love
In them?

Helpful Addresses

Helpful Addresses

BACUP
3 Bath Place
Rivington Street
London, EC2 3JR
Tel: Cancer Information Service Freeline 0800 181199
Cancer Counselling Service 0171 696 9000

BREAST CANCER CARE
Kiln House
210 New Kings Road
London, SW6 4NZ
Tel: Helplines; London 0171 867 1103
Nationwide Freeline 0500 245 345

BRITISH ASSOCIATION FOR COUNSELLING
1 Regent Place
Rugby, CV21 2PJ
Tel: 01788 578328

CANCER CARE SOCIETY
21 Zetland Road
Redland, Bristol
BS6 7AH
Tel: 0117 942 7419

CANCER HELP CENTRE
Grove House
Cornwallis Grove
Clifton, Bristol
BS8 4PG
Tel: 0117 974 3216

CANCERLINK
17 Brittania Street
London, WC1X 9JN
Tel: Cancer Information Service 0171 833 2451
Asian Language Line 0171 713 7867
MAC helpline for young people affected by cancer:
  Freephone 0800 591028

CANCER RELIEF MACMILLAN FUND
Anchor House
15/19 Britten Street
London, SW3 3TZ
Tel: 0171 351 7811

CARERS NATIONAL ASSOCIATION HEAD OFFICE
20-25 Glasshouse Yard
London, EC1A 4JS
Tel: 0171 490 8898

THE COMPASSIONATE FRIENDS
53 North Street
Bristol, BS3 1EN
Tel: 0117 953 9639

CRUSE
Bereavement Care
126 Sheen Road
Richmond, TW9 1UR
Tel: 0181 940 4818
Helpline: 0181 332 7227

HOSPICE INFORMATION SERVICE
St. Christopher's Hospice
51-59 Lawrie Park Road
Sydenham, London
SE26 6DZ
Tel: 0181 778 9252

INSTITUTE FOR COMPLEMENTARY MEDICINE
PO Box 194
London
SE16 1Q2

THE INSTITUTE OF FAMILY THERAPY
43 New Cavendish Street
London
W1M 7RG
Tel: 0171 935 1651

THE MALCOLM SARGENT CANCER FUND FOR
CHILDREN
14 Abingdon Road
London, W8 6AF
Tel: 0171 937 4548

MARIE CURIE CANCER CARE
28 Belgrave Square
London, SW1X 8QG
Tel: 0171 235 3325

THE NATIONAL CANCER ALLIANCE
PO Box 579
Oxford, OX4 1LP
Tel: 01865 793566

THE SUE RYDER FOUNDATION
Cavendish
Sudbury, Suffolk
CO10 8AY
Tel: 01787 280252

WOMEN'S NATIONWIDE CANCER CONTROL
CAMPAIGN
Suna House
128/130 Curtain Road
London, EC2A 3AR
Tel: 0171 729 4688
Helpline 0171 729 2229

Scotland

Breast Cancer Care
13A Castle Terrace
Edinburgh, EH1 2DP
Tel: 0131 221 0407
Suite 2/8 65 Bath Street
Glasgow, G2 2BX
Tel: 0141 353 1050

Cancerlink
9 Castle Terrace
Edinburgh
EH1 2DP
Tel: 0131 228 5557

Cancer Relief Macmillan Fund
9 Castle Terrace
Edinburgh
EH1 2DP
Tel: 0131 229 3276

Wales

The Tenovus Cancer Information Centre
142 Whitchurch Road
Cardiff
CF4 3NA
Tel: (Admin) 01222 619846
Freephone Helpline 0800 526 527

Northern Ireland

The Ulster Cancer Foundation
40-42 Eglantine Avenue
Belfast, BT9 6DX
Tel: 01232 663281/2/3
Helpline 01232 663439

A Page for your own notes: